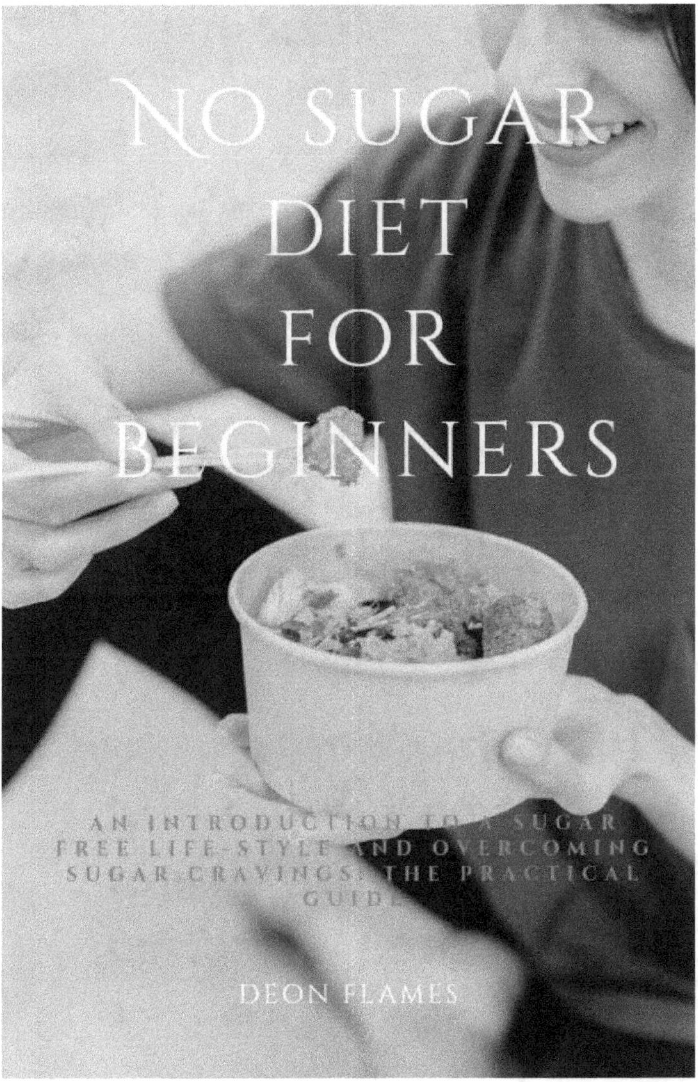

NO SUGAR DIET FOR BEGINNERS

AN INTRODUCTION TO A SUGAR FREE LIFE-STYLE AND OVERCOMING SUGAR CRAVINGS: THE PRACTICAL GUIDE

DEON FLAMES

NO SUGAR DIET FOR BEGINNERS

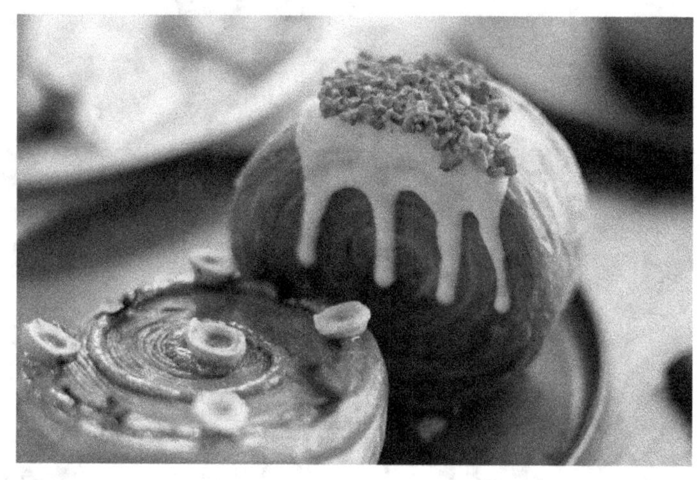

Introduction to a sugar free life-style and overcoming sugar cravings: practical strategies

Deon flames
Copyright © 2023 by Deon flames

All rights reserved. No part of this publication may be reproduced, distributed, or transmitted in any form or by any means, including photocopying, recording, or other electronic or mechanical methods, without the prior written permission of the publisher, except in the case of brief quotations embodied in critical reviews and certain other noncommercial uses permitted by copyright law.

For permission requests, write or contact the publisher below:

Deon flames

deonflames2000@gmail.com

Table of Contents

Introduction

Once upon a time, in a small town, lived Julian, a woman who decided to embark on a sugar-free journey after reading a captivating no-sugar diet book. Motivated by the promise of improved health and well-being, she eagerly embraced a life without the sweet temptations that once ruled her daily menu.

Armed with the knowledge gained from the book, Julian transformed her kitchen, replacing sugary snacks with wholesome alternatives. She explored the world of natural sweeteners and experimented with recipes that allowed her to indulge her taste buds without compromising her commitment.

As days turned into weeks, Julian noticed a remarkable change in her energy levels and overall vitality. She felt more focused and rejuvenated, and her friends began to take notice of her radiant glow. The once daunting journey became a fulfilling adventure, as Emily discovered the joy of nourishing her body with nutritious foods.

Her newfound lifestyle inspired those around her, prompting friends and family to join in her sugar-free quest. Together, they explored local farmers' markets, discovered innovative recipes, and swapped sugar-laden desserts for healthier alternatives.

In time, Julian's story reached the ears of the community, and she found herself leading workshops on sugar-free living. Her journey from reading a no-sugar diet book to becoming a local advocate for healthier lifestyles became a source of inspiration for many.

As the seasons changed, so did the town's perspective on nutrition. Julian's influence led to a shift in local habits, with more people embracing the benefits of a sugar-free existence. The community flourished with newfound energy and well-being, all sparked by one woman's determination to live a healthier life based on the wisdom found in the pages of a simple book.

In the bustling world of nutritional literature, our protagonist embarked on a transformative journey after delving into the pages of a captivating "No Sugar Diet" book. Drawn into the promises of improved health and vitality, they navigated the complexities of sugar-free living, unraveling a narrative that would reshape their relationship with food and redefine their well-being. Join us as we explore the profound impact this literary adventure had on their lifestyle and the lessons it holds for all those seeking a sweeter, yet sugar-free, path to wellness.

Choosing a no-sugar diet offers various health benefits. First, it helps regulate blood sugar levels, reducing the risk of diabetes. Additionally, a sugar-free lifestyle promotes weight management by eliminating empty calories. It can also improve heart health by lowering the risk of cardiovascular diseases linked to excessive sugar intake. Moreover, cutting out sugar supports dental health, reducing the risk of cavities and gum disease. Lastly, a no-sugar diet will enhance mental clarity and reduce fatigue by stabilizing energy levels. Now let's dive into the experience fully.

Sugar is a simple carbohydrate and it plays a significant role in our daily diet and nutrition. It exists in various forms, such as glucose, fructose, and sucrose of which I don't really want to bug you with all of that, and it can be naturally present in foods or added during processing. Understanding sugar involves considering its sources, impact on health, and the importance of moderation.

The World Health Organization (WHO) recommends limiting added sugars to less than 10% of daily caloric intake.
It's crucial to be mindful of hidden sugars in processed foods and beverages.

Simple sugars can lead to rapid spikes in blood sugar levels, especially when consumed without accompanying fiber and protein. Continuous spikes may contribute to insulin resistance and an increased risk of type 2 diabetes.

Understanding sugar content in food involves reading nutrition labels. Look out for various terms like sucrose, fructose, and corn syrup.

Be cautious of products labeled as "low fat" or "diet," as they might compensate with higher sugar content.

Choosing natural sources of sugars, like fruits and honey, can provide sweetness along with additional nutrients.
Opting for whole, unprocessed foods is a simple way to reduce added sugar intake.

Some studies suggest a link between high sugar intake and mental health issues, including increased risk of depression and cognitive decline. However, more research is needed in this area.

Sugar can have addictive qualities, leading to cravings and overconsumption. This can make it challenging for individuals to cut back on sugary foods.

Types of sugar:

Natural Sugars: This type of sugar exists by nature and are mostly found in fruits, vegetables, and dairy products, natural sugars come with fiber, vitamins, and minerals, providing a balanced nutritional package.

Added Sugars: These are sugars added during food processing, often to enhance flavor. Common sources include sugary beverages, snacks, and baked foods.

Impact of sugar on health:

Energy Source: Sugar serves as a quick energy source, especially glucose, which is vital for brain function and overall bodily activities.

Caloric Content: Excessive sugar intake can contribute to weight gain due to its high caloric content. This, in turn, may increase the risk of obesity and related health issues.

Dental Health: Sugars can promote tooth decay as they provide a substrate for bacteria in the mouth to thrive.

Rather than eliminating sugar entirely, moderation is key. Balancing overall caloric intake and being mindful of the types of sugars consumed can contribute to a healthier lifestyle.

In summary, understanding sugar involves recognizing its different forms, considering its impact on health, and making informed choices to maintain a balanced diet. Moderation, along with a focus on natural sources of sugars, is essential for overall well-being.

Chapter 2: Getting Started

It is a widely known and an accepted fact that nutrition is the science/mechanism that explores how the body uses the nutrients found in food for growth, maintenance, as well as overall well-being of the body.

Assessing your current sugar intake

Assessing your current sugar intake is crucial for maintaining a healthy lifestyle. Start by examining food labels to identify added sugars. Look for terms like sucrose, high fructose corn syrup, and other sweeteners. Keep in mind that natural sugars in fruits and dairy are different from added sugars. Evaluate your daily meals and snacks, considering both processed and homemade items. Beverages, such as sodas and sweetened drinks, can contribute significantly to sugar intake. Gradually reduce the consumption of sugary snacks and replace them with healthier alternatives like fruits, nuts, or yogurt. Consider the impact of hidden sugars in seemingly healthy foods like sauces, dressings, and low-fat products. Being aware of these sources helps you make informed choices. Pay attention to portion sizes, as consuming large quantities of even low-sugar foods can add up. Monitor your sugar intake in relation to recommended guidelines. The American Heart Association suggests limiting added sugars to 25 grams (6 teaspoons) for women and 38 grams (9 teaspoons) for men per day. Keep a food diary to track your daily sugar consumption, making it easier to identify patterns and areas for improvement. Assessing your sugar intake also involves recognizing the psychological aspect of cravings. Identify triggers that lead to excessive sugar consumption, such as stress or emotional factors. Develop strategies to cope with these triggers without turning to sugary snacks. Regularly review your dietary choices and adjust as needed. Gradual changes are more sustainable than abrupt restrictions. Consult with a healthcare professional or nutritionist for personalized advice based on your health goals and specific needs. assessing your current sugar intake involves scrutinizing food labels, recognizing hidden sources, monitoring portion sizes, and understanding the psychological aspects of cravings. By being mindful of your sugar consumption, you can make informed choices that contribute to overall.

Setting realistic goals

Setting realistic goals for a no sugar diet is crucial for beginners to ensure long-term success and sustainable lifestyle changes. Here are some key steps to help establish achievable objectives:

Define Clear Objectives:

Clearly outline your reasons for adopting a no sugar diet. Whether it's weight loss, improved energy levels, or overall health, having a specific goal provides motivation.

Understand Sugar Sources:

Educate yourself on different sugar sources, including hidden sugars in processed foods. This awareness will empower you to make informed choices and avoid unnecessary sugar intake.

Gradual Reduction:

Instead of abruptly eliminating all sugar, consider a gradual reduction approach. Start by cutting back on sugary snacks or beverages, allowing your taste buds and habits to adjust over time.

Set Measurable Targets:
Establish measurable goals, such as reducing sugar intake by a certain percentage each week or limiting the number of sugary snacks per day.

Tangible targets make progress more apparent and achievable.

Read Food Labels:
Develop the habit of reading nutrition labels to identify hidden sugars in products. This skill is essential for making informed choices and avoiding unexpected sources of added sugars.

Meal Planning:
Plan your meals ahead of time, focusing on whole, unprocessed foods. This not only helps in avoiding added sugars but also ensures a balanced and nutritious diet.

Hydration Focus:
Emphasize water intake and reduce reliance on sugary beverages. Gradually replace sodas and sugary drinks with water, herbal teas, or infused water for a refreshing alternative.

Celebrate Small Wins:
Acknowledge and celebrate your achievements, no matter how small. Recognizing progress boosts motivation and helps build positive habits.

Mindful Eating:
Practice mindful eating to become more aware of your food choices and to savor the flavors of natural, unsweetened foods. This can help reduce cravings for sugary snacks.

Regular Assessments:
Periodically assess your progress and adjust your goals accordingly. If certain aspects of your no sugar diet are proving difficult, consider revising your approach to make it more attainable.

Be Patient:
Changing dietary habits takes time. Be patient with yourself and understand that setbacks may occur. Use them as learning experiences and continue moving forward.

Chapter 3: The No sugar diet in practice

A no-sugar diet involves avoiding added sugars and focusing on consuming foods with minimal or no sugar content. Approved foods typically include whole, unprocessed foods, while restricted foods are those with added sugars or high natural sugar content. Let's briefly lunch into an extensive overview:

Approved and restricted foods

Approved Foods:

Vegetables: Most vegetables are low in sugar and high in fiber, making them ideal for a no-sugar diet. Leafy greens, broccoli, cauliflower, and bell peppers are excellent choices.

Fruits in Moderation: While some fruits contain natural sugars, they also provide essential nutrients. Opt for berries, avocados, and tomatoes, which have lower sugar content compared to tropical fruits.

Proteins: Lean proteins like poultry, fish, tofu, and legumes are great choices. They help maintain muscle mass and keep you feeling full.

Whole Grains: Choose whole grains like quinoa, brown rice, and oats over refined grains. They offer more nutrients and have a lower impact on blood sugar

Nuts and Seeds: Rich in healthy fats, nuts, and seeds are excellent snacks. However, consume them in moderation due to their calorie density.

Dairy (in moderation): Opt for plain, unsweetened dairy products like Greek yogurt or cheese. Be cautious with flavored yogurts, as they often contain added sugars.

Healthy Fats: Include sources of healthy fats such as avocados, olive oil, and fatty fish like salmon. These fats contribute to overall well-being.

Herbs and Spices: Enhance flavor without added sugars by using herbs and spices in your cooking. They can add variety and depth to your meals.

Restricted foods:

Added Sugars: Avoid foods with added sugars, including sodas, candies, pastries, and sugary beverages. Check food labels for hidden sugars under various names like sucrose, high fructose corn syrup, or agave nectar.

Processed Foods: Many processed foods contain hidden sugars. Be cautious with packaged snacks, sauces, and dressings. Opt for whole, unprocessed alternatives whenever possible.

White Flour Products: Refined carbohydrates like white bread, pasta, and baked goods can spike blood sugar levels. Choose whole-grain options instead.

Sweetened Beverages: Sugary drinks like sodas, energy drinks, and fruit juices are high in added sugars. Opt for water, herbal teas, or unsweetened beverages.

Sweetened Dairy: Flavored yogurts, ice creams, and sweetened milk alternatives often contain added sugars. Choose plain, unsweetened options and add natural sweetness with fruits if desired.

Processed Meats: Some processed meats may have added sugars in their seasoning or curing process. Choose fresh, lean meats and prepare them at home.

Condiments with Added Sugars: Check labels for condiments like ketchup, barbecue sauce, and salad dressings, as they often contain hidden sugars. Look for sugar-free or make your own at home.

Remember, consulting with a healthcare professional or nutritionist is advisable before making significant changes to your diet, especially if you have specific health concerns or conditions.

Meal planning and recipes

Meal planning for a no-sugar diet is crucial to ensure a balanced and satisfying culinary experience while avoiding added sugars. Here's a comprehensive guide to get beginners started:

Breakfast:
Avocado and Egg Breakfast Bowl:
Top a bowl of scrambled eggs with sliced avocado, cherry tomatoes, and a sprinkle of herbs.

Greek Yogurt Parfait:
Layer Greek yogurt with fresh berries, nuts, and a drizzle of natural honey for sweetness.

Lunch:
Grilled Chicken Salad:

Combine grilled chicken breast with mixed greens, cherry tomatoes, cucumber, and a light vinaigrette.
Quinoa and Vegetable Stir-Fry:

Stir-fry colorful vegetables with quinoa and tofu or shrimp, seasoned with soy sauce and ginger.

Dinner:
Baked Salmon with Lemon and Herbs:
Season salmon fillets with lemon, garlic, and herbs, then bake until flaky.
Zucchini Noodles with Pesto:
Spiralize zucchini into noodles and toss with homemade basil pesto for a satisfying pasta alternative.
Snacks:
Crudité Platter with Hummus:
Enjoy a variety of raw veggies with a side of hummus for a crunchy and satisfying snack.
Nuts and Seeds Mix:
Create a mix of almonds, walnuts, and pumpkin seeds for a nutrient-dense snack.
Dessert:
Berry Sorbet:
Blend frozen berries with a splash of coconut water for a refreshing and sugar-free sorbet.
Dark Chocolate Dipped Strawberries:
Dip fresh strawberries in melted dark chocolate for a sweet treat with minimal sugar.

Hydration:
Infused Water:
Enhance your water with slices of cucumber,
lemon, and mint for added flavor without added
sugars.
Remember, adapting to a no-sugar diet is a gradual
process. Experiment with these recipes, listen to
your body, and feel free to customize meals based
on personal preferences. Always consult with a
healthcare professional or nutritionist for
personalized advice.

Chapter 4: Overcoming challenges and monitoring progress

Dealing with sugar cravings can be quite
challenging and tough, but here are strategies to
help manage them effectively.

Understand the Trigger:
Identify the triggers that lead to your sugar
cravings. Stress, boredom, or emotional factors can
often play a role. Once you recognize these
triggers, you can work on addressing them directly.

Stay Hydrated:
Sometimes, dehydration can be mistaken for hunger or sugar cravings. Ensure you're adequately hydrated throughout the day by drinking water regularly.

Balanced Meals:
Consume balanced meals that include a mix of proteins, healthy fats, and complex carbohydrates. This helps stabilize blood sugar levels and reduces the likelihood of intense cravings.

Gradual Reduction:
If you're used to a high-sugar diet, consider gradually reducing your sugar intake instead of going cold turkey. This can make the transition more manageable.

Choose Whole Foods:
Opt for whole, unprocessed foods. Fruits, vegetables, lean proteins, and whole grains can provide essential nutrients and fiber, helping to keep you full and satisfied.

Healthy Snacking:
Have healthy snacks on hand to combat sudden cravings. Nuts, seeds, and Greek yogurt with berries are nutritious options that can curb your sweet tooth.

Mindful Eating:

Practice mindful eating by paying attention to the flavors, textures, and satisfaction derived from each bite. This can enhance your awareness of what you eat and reduce impulsive sugar consumption.

Get Moving:

Engage in regular physical activity. Exercise can improve mood, reduce stress, and naturally decrease cravings by releasing endorphins.

Adequate Sleep:

Ensure you get enough quality sleep. Lack of sleep can disrupt hormonal balance and increase cravings for sugary foods.

Substitute Smartly:

Experiment with healthier sweeteners like stevia or monk fruit as alternatives to refined sugars. Be cautious not to overuse substitutes, though.

Plan Ahead:

Plan your meals and snacks in advance. Having healthy options readily available reduces the likelihood of succumbing to sugary temptations.

Support System:

Share your goal with friends or family. Having a support system can provide encouragement and understanding during challenging moments.

Reward Yourself:

Celebrate your achievements, whether big or small. Recognizing your progress can boost motivation and make the journey more rewarding.

Professional Guidance:
If needed, consult with a nutritionist or healthcare professional to create a personalized plan tailored to your specific needs and challenges.

Remember, overcoming sugar cravings is a gradual process that involves lifestyle changes. Be patient with yourself, stay committed to your goals, and celebrate the positive changes you make along the way.

Please note that there are quite a lot withdrawal symptoms and challenges you are going to meet which are temporary, and as your body adjusts to a no-sugar diet, the cravings and discomfort should subside.

Staying Motivated

Staying motivated on a no-sugar diet can be challenging but rewarding. Start by setting realistic goals and celebrating small victories. Educate yourself about hidden sugars in food, and plan nutritious meals to avoid cravings. Surround yourself with a supportive community or partner to share the journey. Keep healthy snacks on hand to curb sweet cravings, and experiment with natural sweeteners like stevia or monk fruit. Track your progress, stay focused on the benefits, and remember that it's okay to indulge occasionally in moderation. Consistency and a positive mindset are key to long-term success.

Monitoring progress

To monitor progress on a no-sugar diet for beginners, track your daily food intake, noting any sources of added sugars. Use a food diary or apps like MyFitnessPal or any related app. Regularly check labels for hidden sugars, and focus on whole, unprocessed foods. Monitor energy levels, mood, and cravings to gauge the impact of reduced sugar intake. Keep track of weight, measurements, and overall well-being. Periodically reassess goals and celebrate small victories to stay motivated on your sugar-free journey.

Chapter 5: Long-term maintenance

HiLong-term maintenance in a no sugar diet for beginners involves establishing sustainable habits and making gradual lifestyle changes. Focus on whole, unprocessed foods, incorporate a variety of nutrients, and be mindful of hidden sugars in packaged items. Stay hydrated, prioritize balanced meals, and experiment with sugar alternatives if needed. Regularly monitor your progress, celebrate small victories, and seek support from peers or professionals to stay motivated. Remember, consistency and patience are key in adapting to a sustainable no sugar lifestyle.

Building sustainable habits

Start by gradually reducing added sugars in your diet, replacing sugary snacks with healthier options like fruits or nuts.

Educate yourself about hidden sugars in processed foods, read labels, and make informed choices to minimize sugar intake.

Create a meal plan with balanced, whole foods to ensure you're getting essential nutrients without relying on sugary items.

Stay hydrated to curb sugar cravings, as sometimes thirst can be mistaken for hunger.

Incorporate more fiber-rich foods into your diet, as they can help stabilize blood sugar levels and keep you feeling full.

Establish a consistent eating schedule to regulate blood sugar and prevent mindless snacking.

Find enjoyable sugar-free alternatives for your favorite treats to satisfy cravings without compromising your commitment.

Build a support system or join a community with individuals pursuing a no-sugar lifestyle for motivation and shared experiences.

Celebrate small victories and be patient with yourself during the transition to a no-sugar diet.

Finding balance in a no sugar conscious lifestyle

Balancing a no-sugar lifestyle involves mindful choices and awareness. Focus on whole foods like fruits, vegetables, and lean proteins, and experiment with natural sweeteners. Stay hydrated, plan meals ahead, and gradually reduce added sugars to avoid feeling deprived. Listen to your body's signals and celebrate small victories, fostering a sustainable and balanced approach to a sugar-conscious life.

Maintaining overall well-being

When embarking on a no-sugar diet, focus on whole, unprocessed foods like fruits, vegetables, lean proteins, and whole grains. Stay hydrated, prioritize fiber-rich foods, and be mindful of hidden sugars in sauces and processed items. Gradually reduce sugar intake to ease the transition, and consider healthy alternatives like stevia or monk fruit. Monitor energy levels, prioritize adequate sleep, and engage in regular physical activity to support overall well-being. Consult a healthcare professional for personalized advice.

• Conclusion

In conclusion, embarking on a no sugar diet journey as a beginner is a transformative and empowering experience. This comprehensive guide has equipped you with the knowledge and practical tips needed to navigate the challenges of eliminating added sugars from your life. By embracing whole, nutrient-dense foods and adopting mindful eating habits, you've taken a significant step towards improved physical health and mental well-being.

As you close the pages of this book, remember that the journey to a sugar-free lifestyle is a gradual process, and success lies in consistency and perseverance. Celebrate the small victories, whether it's resisting a tempting dessert or discovering new, delicious sugar-free recipes. Recognize the positive changes in your energy levels, mood, and overall health as you distance yourself from the detrimental effects of excessive sugar consumption.

This guide has not only provided you with practical strategies but also emphasized the importance of a supportive environment and a positive mindset. As you navigate social situations and potential setbacks, remember that you have the tools to make informed choices and prioritize your health.

In the broader context, adopting a no sugar lifestyle extends beyond personal benefits—it contributes to a healthier society by reducing the burden of sugar-related health issues. By sharing your knowledge and experiences, you can inspire others to embark on their own sugar-free journey.

In essence, this book serves as a foundation for a sustainable and fulfilling no sugar lifestyle. Armed with newfound awareness and a commitment to a healthier future, you are ready to embrace the rewards of a life free from the shackles of excessive sugar consumption. May your journey be filled with vitality, joy, and the countless benefits that come with prioritizing your well-being.